Powerlifting Training Log

Robert L. Dunn

Powerlifting Training Log
© 2018 Robert L. Dunn.

ISBN: 9781729407851

DISCLAIMER:

The Author recommends that you consult with your physician before beginning any exercise program. You should be in good physical condition and be able to participate in the exercise. The Author is not a licensed medical care provider and represents that he has no expertise in diagnosing, examining, or treating medical conditions of any kind, or in determining the effect of any specific exercise on a medical condition. You should understand that when participating in any exercise or exercise program, there is the possibility of physical injury. If you engage in this exercise or exercise program, you agree that you do so at your own risk, are voluntarily participating in these activities, and assume all risk of injury to yourself.

CONTENTS:

Introduction

Powerlifting Training Log Entries

REFERENCE SECTION:

HOW TO DOCUMENT WORKOUTS IN THIS BOOK:

SAMPLE WORKOUT 1

SAMPLE WORKOUT 2

SAMPLE CONTEST LOG ENTRIES

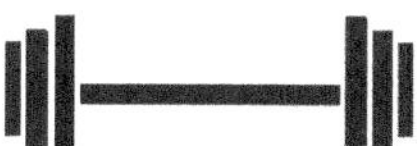

Contest Log Entries

Introduction

I grew up in Struthers, Ohio, and I began training with weights at the age of 13. My older brother, Jerry, paved the way for me as I watched him training in our basement a few years earlier. He made great strides in size and strength and developed an incredible physique by the age of 15.

While using what would be considered primitive equipment by today's standards, I also made great strides. I spent many hours at the Youngstown YMCA training with my good friend, George Garchar, who went on to have a stellar powerlifting career as a teenager.

I entered my first powerlifting meet at the age of 15 and gradually became nationally competitive at the teenage level. My best lift was the deadlift where I eventually pulled 570 in competition at the age of 18. I also ventured into bodybuilding and Olympic lifting and competed up until my early 20's. None of these positive experiences in my formative years would have been possible without the love and support of the wonderful parents with whom my brother and I were blessed.

After a long hiatus from the iron game, I got serious about running and competing in road races. I ran as long as my knees would permit and eventually rediscovered powerlifting in my 50's. I have been actively involved and enjoying the sport more than ever.

I hope this log will make it easy and efficient to track workouts and record progress made in training. I have also included a section for you to keep an accurate record of competitions entered.

The three common lifts (squat, bench press and deadlift) are listed along with the curl which is a competitive lift in the 100% RAW Powerlifting Federation.

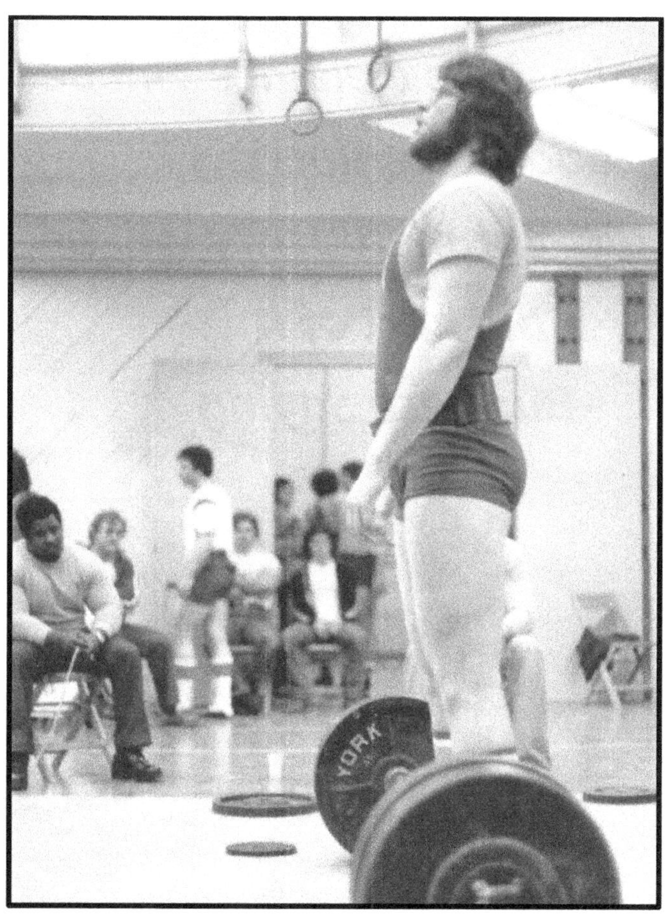

*Who aims at excellence will be
above mediocrity;
who aims at mediocrity will be
far short of it.*
–Burmese Saying

DATE: _______ PLACE:______________________ WEIGHT:_______

EXERCISE		SET 1	SET 2	SET 3	SET 4	SET 5	SET 6	SET 7
SQUAT	REPS							
	WEIGHT							
BENCH PRESS	REPS							
	WEIGHT							
DEADLIFT	REPS							
	WEIGHT							
CURL	REPS							
	WEIGHT							

ASSISTANCE EXERCISES		SET 1	SET 2	SET 3	SET 4	SET 5
	REPS					
	WEIGHT					
	REPS					
	WEIGHT					
	REPS					
	WEIGHT					
	REPS					
	WEIGHT					

COMMENTS / GOALS / SUPPLEMENTS USED

"Ordinary people have always accomplished extraordinary things, be one of them." –Robert L. Dunn

DATE: ________ PLACE:______________________ WEIGHT:_______

EXERCISE		SET 1	SET 2	SET 3	SET 4	SET 5	SET 6	SET 7
SQUAT	REPS							
	WEIGHT							
BENCH PRESS	REPS							
	WEIGHT							
DEADLIFT	REPS							
	WEIGHT							
CURL	REPS							
	WEIGHT							

ASSISTANCE EXERCISES		SET 1	SET 2	SET 3	SET 4	SET 5
	REPS					
	WEIGHT					
	REPS					
	WEIGHT					
	REPS					
	WEIGHT					
	REPS					
	WEIGHT					

COMMENTS / GOALS / SUPPLEMENTS USED

"Nothing is impossible, the word itself says, 'I'm possible.'"
–Katherine Hepburn

DATE: _______   PLACE:___________________ WEIGHT:_______

EXERCISE		SET 1	SET 2	SET 3	SET 4	SET 5	SET 6	SET 7
SQUAT	REPS							
	WEIGHT							
BENCH PRESS	REPS							
	WEIGHT							
DEADLIFT	REPS							
	WEIGHT							
CURL	REPS							
	WEIGHT							

ASSISTANCE EXERCISES		SET 1	SET 2	SET 3	SET 4	SET 5
	REPS					
	WEIGHT					
	REPS					
	WEIGHT					
	REPS					
	WEIGHT					
	REPS					
	WEIGHT					

COMMENTS / GOALS / SUPPLEMENTS USED

"POWER = Passion. Optimism. Work. Endure. Reward."
-Robert L. Dunn

DATE: _______   PLACE:____________________   WEIGHT:_______

EXERCISE		SET 1	SET 2	SET 3	SET 4	SET 5	SET 6	SET 7
SQUAT	REPS							
	WEIGHT							
BENCH PRESS	REPS							
	WEIGHT							
DEADLIFT	REPS							
	WEIGHT							
CURL	REPS							
	WEIGHT							

ASSISTANCE EXERCISES		SET 1	SET 2	SET 3	SET 4	SET 5
	REPS					
	WEIGHT					
	REPS					
	WEIGHT					
	REPS					
	WEIGHT					
	REPS					
	WEIGHT					

COMMENTS / GOALS / SUPPLEMENTS USED

"With self-discipline most anything is possible."
-Theodore Roosevelt

DATE: _______   PLACE:____________________ WEIGHT:_______

EXERCISE		SET 1	SET 2	SET 3	SET 4	SET 5	SET 6	SET 7
SQUAT	REPS							
	WEIGHT							
BENCH PRESS	REPS							
	WEIGHT							
DEADLIFT	REPS							
	WEIGHT							
CURL	REPS							
	WEIGHT							

ASSISTANCE EXERCISES		SET 1	SET 2	SET 3	SET 4	SET 5
	REPS					
	WEIGHT					
	REPS					
	WEIGHT					
	REPS					
	WEIGHT					
	REPS					
	WEIGHT					

COMMENTS / GOALS / SUPPLEMENTS USED

"Quality is not an act, it is a habit." -Aristotle

DATE: _______ PLACE:_____________________ WEIGHT:_______

EXERCISE		SET 1	SET 2	SET 3	SET 4	SET 5	SET 6	SET 7
SQUAT	REPS							
	WEIGHT							
BENCH PRESS	REPS							
	WEIGHT							
DEADLIFT	REPS							
	WEIGHT							
CURL	REPS							
	WEIGHT							

ASSISTANCE EXERCISES		SET 1	SET 2	SET 3	SET 4	SET 5
	REPS					
	WEIGHT					
	REPS					
	WEIGHT					
	REPS					
	WEIGHT					
	REPS					
	WEIGHT					

COMMENTS / GOALS / SUPPLEMENTS USED

"Do something wonderful, people may imitate it."
-Albert Schweitzer

DATE: ________   PLACE: ______________________   WEIGHT: _______

EXERCISE		SET 1	SET 2	SET 3	SET 4	SET 5	SET 6	SET 7
SQUAT	REPS							
	WEIGHT							
BENCH PRESS	REPS							
	WEIGHT							
DEADLIFT	REPS							
	WEIGHT							
CURL	REPS							
	WEIGHT							

ASSISTANCE EXERCISES		SET 1	SET 2	SET 3	SET 4	SET 5
	REPS					
	WEIGHT					
	REPS					
	WEIGHT					
	REPS					
	WEIGHT					
	REPS					
	WEIGHT					

COMMENTS / GOALS / SUPPLEMENTS USED

"When your brother is down, say something positive to lift him up." -Robert L. Dunn

DATE: _______ PLACE:___________________ WEIGHT:_______

EXERCISE		SET 1	SET 2	SET 3	SET 4	SET 5	SET 6	SET 7
SQUAT	REPS							
	WEIGHT							
BENCH PRESS	REPS							
	WEIGHT							
DEADLIFT	REPS							
	WEIGHT							
CURL	REPS							
	WEIGHT							

ASSISTANCE EXERCISES		SET 1	SET 2	SET 3	SET 4	SET 5
	REPS					
	WEIGHT					
	REPS					
	WEIGHT					
	REPS					
	WEIGHT					
	REPS					
	WEIGHT					

COMMENTS / GOALS / SUPPLEMENTS USED

"Your age is a number, don't let it limit you."
-Robert L. Dunn

DATE: _______   PLACE:_____________________ WEIGHT:_______

EXERCISE		SET 1	SET 2	SET 3	SET 4	SET 5	SET 6	SET 7
SQUAT	REPS							
	WEIGHT							
BENCH PRESS	REPS							
	WEIGHT							
DEADLIFT	REPS							
	WEIGHT							
CURL	REPS							
	WEIGHT							

ASSISTANCE EXERCISES		SET 1	SET 2	SET 3	SET 4	SET 5
	REPS					
	WEIGHT					
	REPS					
	WEIGHT					
	REPS					
	WEIGHT					
	REPS					
	WEIGHT					

COMMENTS / GOALS / SUPPLEMENTS USED

"Get action, seize the moment, man was never intended to become an oyster." –Theodore Roosevelt

DATE: _______   PLACE:____________________   WEIGHT:_______

EXERCISE		SET 1	SET 2	SET 3	SET 4	SET 5	SET 6	SET 7
SQUAT	REPS							
	WEIGHT							
BENCH PRESS	REPS							
	WEIGHT							
DEADLIFT	REPS							
	WEIGHT							
CURL	REPS							
	WEIGHT							

ASSISTANCE EXERCISES		SET 1	SET 2	SET 3	SET 4	SET 5
	REPS					
	WEIGHT					
	REPS					
	WEIGHT					
	REPS					
	WEIGHT					
	REPS					
	WEIGHT					

COMMENTS / GOALS / SUPPLEMENTS USED

"Go for it now, the future is promised to no one."
—Wayne Dyer

DATE: ________   PLACE: _____________________ WEIGHT: _______

EXERCISE		SET 1	SET 2	SET 3	SET 4	SET 5	SET 6	SET 7
SQUAT	REPS							
	WEIGHT							
BENCH PRESS	REPS							
	WEIGHT							
DEADLIFT	REPS							
	WEIGHT							
CURL	REPS							
	WEIGHT							

ASSISTANCE EXERCISES		SET 1	SET 2	SET 3	SET 4	SET 5
	REPS					
	WEIGHT					
	REPS					
	WEIGHT					
	REPS					
	WEIGHT					
	REPS					
	WEIGHT					

COMMENTS / GOALS / SUPPLEMENTS USED

"The secret of getting ahead is getting started."
-Mark Twain

DATE: _______ PLACE:____________________ WEIGHT:_______

EXERCISE		SET 1	SET 2	SET 3	SET 4	SET 5	SET 6	SET 7
SQUAT	REPS							
	WEIGHT							
BENCH PRESS	REPS							
	WEIGHT							
DEADLIFT	REPS							
	WEIGHT							
CURL	REPS							
	WEIGHT							

ASSISTANCE EXERCISES		SET 1	SET 2	SET 3	SET 4	SET 5
	REPS					
	WEIGHT					
	REPS					
	WEIGHT					
	REPS					
	WEIGHT					
	REPS					
	WEIGHT					

COMMENTS / GOALS / SUPPLEMENTS USED

"Well done is better than well said."
-Benjamin Franklin

DATE: _______   PLACE:_____________________ WEIGHT:_______

EXERCISE		SET 1	SET 2	SET 3	SET 4	SET 5	SET 6	SET 7
SQUAT	REPS							
	WEIGHT							
BENCH	REPS							
PRESS	WEIGHT							
DEADLIFT	REPS							
	WEIGHT							
CURL	REPS							
	WEIGHT							

ASSISTANCE EXERCISES		SET 1	SET 2	SET 3	SET 4	SET 5
	REPS					
	WEIGHT					
	REPS					
	WEIGHT					
	REPS					
	WEIGHT					
	REPS					
	WEIGHT					

COMMENTS / GOALS / SUPPLEMENTS USED

"FEAR: False Evidence Appearing Real"
-Neale Donald Walsch

DATE: _______   PLACE:_____________________   WEIGHT:_______

EXERCISE		SET 1	SET 2	SET 3	SET 4	SET 5	SET 6	SET 7
SQUAT	REPS							
	WEIGHT							
BENCH PRESS	REPS							
	WEIGHT							
DEADLIFT	REPS							
	WEIGHT							
CURL	REPS							
	WEIGHT							

ASSISTANCE EXERCISES		SET 1	SET 2	SET 3	SET 4	SET 5
	REPS					
	WEIGHT					
	REPS					
	WEIGHT					
	REPS					
	WEIGHT					
	REPS					
	WEIGHT					

COMMENTS / GOALS / SUPPLEMENTS USED

"Waste a day, waste an opportunity."
-Robert L. Dunn

DATE: _______   PLACE:____________________   WEIGHT:_______

EXERCISE		SET 1	SET 2	SET 3	SET 4	SET 5	SET 6	SET 7
SQUAT	REPS							
	WEIGHT							
BENCH PRESS	REPS							
	WEIGHT							
DEADLIFT	REPS							
	WEIGHT							
CURL	REPS							
	WEIGHT							

ASSISTANCE EXERCISES		SET 1	SET 2	SET 3	SET 4	SET 5
	REPS					
	WEIGHT					
	REPS					
	WEIGHT					
	REPS					
	WEIGHT					
	REPS					
	WEIGHT					

COMMENTS / GOALS / SUPPLEMENTS USED

"The will to do, the soul to dare, is yours for the taking, if you prepare." –Sir Walter Scott

DATE: _______ PLACE:____________________ WEIGHT:_______

EXERCISE		SET 1	SET 2	SET 3	SET 4	SET 5	SET 6	SET 7
SQUAT	REPS							
	WEIGHT							
BENCH PRESS	REPS							
	WEIGHT							
DEADLIFT	REPS							
	WEIGHT							
CURL	REPS							
	WEIGHT							

ASSISTANCE EXERCISES		SET 1	SET 2	SET 3	SET 4	SET 5
	REPS					
	WEIGHT					
	REPS					
	WEIGHT					
	REPS					
	WEIGHT					
	REPS					
	WEIGHT					

COMMENTS / GOALS / SUPPLEMENTS USED

"Hold fast to dreams, for if dreams die, life is like a broken winged bird that cannot fly." –Langston Hughes

DATE: _______   PLACE:_____________________ WEIGHT:_______

EXERCISE		SET 1	SET 2	SET 3	SET 4	SET 5	SET 6	SET 7
SQUAT	REPS							
	WEIGHT							
BENCH	REPS							
PRESS	WEIGHT							
DEADLIFT	REPS							
	WEIGHT							
CURL	REPS							
	WEIGHT							

ASSISTANCE EXERCISES		SET 1	SET 2	SET 3	SET 4	SET 5
	REPS					
	WEIGHT					
	REPS					
	WEIGHT					
	REPS					
	WEIGHT					
	REPS					
	WEIGHT					

COMMENTS / GOALS / SUPPLEMENTS USED

"Success is getting up just one more time than you fall."
-Oliver Goldsmith

DATE: _______ PLACE:___________________________ WEIGHT:_______

EXERCISE		SET 1	SET 2	SET 3	SET 4	SET 5	SET 6	SET 7
SQUAT	REPS							
	WEIGHT							
BENCH PRESS	REPS							
	WEIGHT							
DEADLIFT	REPS							
	WEIGHT							
CURL	REPS							
	WEIGHT							

ASSISTANCE EXERCISES		SET 1	SET 2	SET 3	SET 4	SET 5
	REPS					
	WEIGHT					
	REPS					
	WEIGHT					
	REPS					
	WEIGHT					
	REPS					
	WEIGHT					

COMMENTS / GOALS / SUPPLEMENTS USED

*"Look for the dream that keeps coming back.
It is your destiny." -Unknown*

DATE: _______   PLACE: _____________________ WEIGHT: _______

EXERCISE		SET 1	SET 2	SET 3	SET 4	SET 5	SET 6	SET 7
SQUAT	REPS							
	WEIGHT							
BENCH PRESS	REPS							
	WEIGHT							
DEADLIFT	REPS							
	WEIGHT							
CURL	REPS							
	WEIGHT							

ASSISTANCE EXERCISES		SET 1	SET 2	SET 3	SET 4	SET 5
	REPS					
	WEIGHT					
	REPS					
	WEIGHT					
	REPS					
	WEIGHT					
	REPS					
	WEIGHT					

COMMENTS / GOALS / SUPPLEMENTS USED

"Don't let negative thinking keep you on the sidelines of life." –Robert L. Dunn

DATE: _______   PLACE:___________________ WEIGHT:______

EXERCISE		SET 1	SET 2	SET 3	SET 4	SET 5	SET 6	SET 7
SQUAT	REPS							
	WEIGHT							
BENCH PRESS	REPS							
	WEIGHT							
DEADLIFT	REPS							
	WEIGHT							
CURL	REPS							
	WEIGHT							

ASSISTANCE EXERCISES		SET 1	SET 2	SET 3	SET 4	SET 5
	REPS					
	WEIGHT					
	REPS					
	WEIGHT					
	REPS					
	WEIGHT					
	REPS					
	WEIGHT					

COMMENTS / GOALS / SUPPLEMENTS USED

"Be ordinary and stay on the couch flipping channels; be extraordinary, put down the bag of chips and move."
-Robert L. Dunn

DATE: _______   PLACE:_____________________ WEIGHT:_______

EXERCISE		SET 1	SET 2	SET 3	SET 4	SET 5	SET 6	SET 7
SQUAT	REPS							
	WEIGHT							
BENCH PRESS	REPS							
	WEIGHT							
DEADLIFT	REPS							
	WEIGHT							
CURL	REPS							
	WEIGHT							

ASSISTANCE EXERCISES		SET 1	SET 2	SET 3	SET 4	SET 5
	REPS					
	WEIGHT					
	REPS					
	WEIGHT					
	REPS					
	WEIGHT					
	REPS					
	WEIGHT					

COMMENTS / GOALS / SUPPLEMENTS USED

"Success is best measured by living up to one's potential."
-Robert L. Dunn

DATE: _______   PLACE:_____________________ WEIGHT:________

EXERCISE		SET 1	SET 2	SET 3	SET 4	SET 5	SET 6	SET 7
SQUAT	REPS							
	WEIGHT							
BENCH	REPS							
PRESS	WEIGHT							
DEADLIFT	REPS							
	WEIGHT							
CURL	REPS							
	WEIGHT							

ASSISTANCE EXERCISES		SET 1	SET 2	SET 3	SET 4	SET 5
	REPS					
	WEIGHT					
	REPS					
	WEIGHT					
	REPS					
	WEIGHT					
	REPS					
	WEIGHT					

COMMENTS / GOALS / SUPPLEMENTS USED

"Ask yourself, how successful are the naysayers who discourage you? –Robert L. Dunn

DATE: _______   PLACE:___________________ WEIGHT:_______

EXERCISE		SET 1	SET 2	SET 3	SET 4	SET 5	SET 6	SET 7
SQUAT	REPS							
	WEIGHT							
BENCH PRESS	REPS							
	WEIGHT							
DEADLIFT	REPS							
	WEIGHT							
CURL	REPS							
	WEIGHT							

ASSISTANCE EXERCISES		SET 1	SET 2	SET 3	SET 4	SET 5
	REPS					
	WEIGHT					
	REPS					
	WEIGHT					
	REPS					
	WEIGHT					
	REPS					
	WEIGHT					

COMMENTS / GOALS / SUPPLEMENTS USED

"Strength is the product of struggle, you must do what others don't to achieve what others won't."
-Henry Rollins

DATE: ______   PLACE:__________________ WEIGHT:______

EXERCISE		SET 1	SET 2	SET 3	SET 4	SET 5	SET 6	SET 7
SQUAT	REPS							
	WEIGHT							
BENCH PRESS	REPS							
	WEIGHT							
DEADLIFT	REPS							
	WEIGHT							
CURL	REPS							
	WEIGHT							

ASSISTANCE EXERCISES		SET 1	SET 2	SET 3	SET 4	SET 5
	REPS					
	WEIGHT					
	REPS					
	WEIGHT					
	REPS					
	WEIGHT					
	REPS					
	WEIGHT					

COMMENTS / GOALS / SUPPLEMENTS USED

"Rest not. Life is sweeping by; go and dare before you die. Something mighty and sublime, leave behind to conquer time." –Johann Wolfgang Von Goethe

DATE: _______   PLACE:___________________ WEIGHT:_______

EXERCISE		SET 1	SET 2	SET 3	SET 4	SET 5	SET 6	SET 7
SQUAT	REPS							
	WEIGHT							
BENCH PRESS	REPS							
	WEIGHT							
DEADLIFT	REPS							
	WEIGHT							
CURL	REPS							
	WEIGHT							

ASSISTANCE EXERCISES		SET 1	SET 2	SET 3	SET 4	SET 5
	REPS					
	WEIGHT					
	REPS					
	WEIGHT					
	REPS					
	WEIGHT					
	REPS					
	WEIGHT					

COMMENTS / GOALS / SUPPLEMENTS USED

"Freedom allows you the opportunity to fulfill your destiny."
-Robert L. Dunn

DATE: _______   PLACE:_____________________ WEIGHT:_______

EXERCISE		SET 1	SET 2	SET 3	SET 4	SET 5	SET 6	SET 7
SQUAT	REPS							
	WEIGHT							
BENCH PRESS	REPS							
	WEIGHT							
DEADLIFT	REPS							
	WEIGHT							
CURL	REPS							
	WEIGHT							

ASSISTANCE EXERCISES		SET 1	SET 2	SET 3	SET 4	SET 5
	REPS					
	WEIGHT					
	REPS					
	WEIGHT					
	REPS					
	WEIGHT					
	REPS					
	WEIGHT					

COMMENTS / GOALS / SUPPLEMENTS USED

"When you arise in the morning, think of what a privilege it is to be alive, to think, to enjoy, to love." –Marcus Aurelius

DATE: _______   PLACE: ____________________ WEIGHT: _______

EXERCISE		SET 1	SET 2	SET 3	SET 4	SET 5	SET 6	SET 7
SQUAT	REPS							
	WEIGHT							
BENCH PRESS	REPS							
	WEIGHT							
DEADLIFT	REPS							
	WEIGHT							
CURL	REPS							
	WEIGHT							

ASSISTANCE EXERCISES		SET 1	SET 2	SET 3	SET 4	SET 5
	REPS					
	WEIGHT					
	REPS					
	WEIGHT					
	REPS					
	WEIGHT					
	REPS					
	WEIGHT					

COMMENTS / GOALS / SUPPLEMENTS USED

"It is never too late to be what you might have been."
–George Eliot

DATE: ________   PLACE:______________________ WEIGHT:_______

EXERCISE		SET 1	SET 2	SET 3	SET 4	SET 5	SET 6	SET 7
SQUAT	REPS							
	WEIGHT							
BENCH PRESS	REPS							
	WEIGHT							
DEADLIFT	REPS							
	WEIGHT							
CURL	REPS							
	WEIGHT							

ASSISTANCE EXERCISES		SET 1	SET 2	SET 3	SET 4	SET 5
	REPS					
	WEIGHT					
	REPS					
	WEIGHT					
	REPS					
	WEIGHT					
	REPS					
	WEIGHT					

COMMENTS / GOALS / SUPPLEMENTS USED

"It takes courage to push yourself to places that you have never been before...to test your limits...to break through barriers. And the day came when the risk it took to remain tight inside the bud was more painful than the risk it took to blossom." –Anais Nin

DATE: _______   PLACE:_____________________ WEIGHT:_______

EXERCISE		SET 1	SET 2	SET 3	SET 4	SET 5	SET 6	SET 7
SQUAT	REPS							
	WEIGHT							
BENCH	REPS							
PRESS	WEIGHT							
DEADLIFT	REPS							
	WEIGHT							
CURL	REPS							
	WEIGHT							

ASSISTANCE EXERCISES		SET 1	SET 2	SET 3	SET 4	SET 5
	REPS					
	WEIGHT					
	REPS					
	WEIGHT					
	REPS					
	WEIGHT					
	REPS					
	WEIGHT					

COMMENTS / GOALS / SUPPLEMENTS USED

"You must do the things you think you cannot do."
-Eleanor Roosevelt

DATE: _______   PLACE:_____________________ WEIGHT:_______

EXERCISE		SET 1	SET 2	SET 3	SET 4	SET 5	SET 6	SET 7
SQUAT	REPS							
	WEIGHT							
BENCH	REPS							
PRESS	WEIGHT							
DEADLIFT	REPS							
	WEIGHT							
CURL	REPS							
	WEIGHT							

ASSISTANCE EXERCISES		SET 1	SET 2	SET 3	SET 4	SET 5
	REPS					
	WEIGHT					
	REPS					
	WEIGHT					
	REPS					
	WEIGHT					
	REPS					
	WEIGHT					

COMMENTS / GOALS / SUPPLEMENTS USED

"There is no time for ease and comfort.
It is time to dare and endure." Winston Churchill

DATE: _______   PLACE: ___________________ WEIGHT: _______

EXERCISE		SET 1	SET 2	SET 3	SET 4	SET 5	SET 6	SET 7
SQUAT	REPS							
	WEIGHT							
BENCH PRESS	REPS							
	WEIGHT							
DEADLIFT	REPS							
	WEIGHT							
CURL	REPS							
	WEIGHT							

ASSISTANCE EXERCISES		SET 1	SET 2	SET 3	SET 4	SET 5
	REPS					
	WEIGHT					
	REPS					
	WEIGHT					
	REPS					
	WEIGHT					
	REPS					
	WEIGHT					

COMMENTS / GOALS / SUPPLEMENTS USED

"He gives strength to the weary and increases the power of the weak." Isaiah 40:29 (NIV)

DATE: _______   PLACE:____________________ WEIGHT:_______

EXERCISE		SET 1	SET 2	SET 3	SET 4	SET 5	SET 6	SET 7
SQUAT	REPS							
	WEIGHT							
BENCH PRESS	REPS							
	WEIGHT							
DEADLIFT	REPS							
	WEIGHT							
CURL	REPS							
	WEIGHT							

ASSISTANCE EXERCISES		SET 1	SET 2	SET 3	SET 4	SET 5
	REPS					
	WEIGHT					
	REPS					
	WEIGHT					
	REPS					
	WEIGHT					
	REPS					
	WEIGHT					

COMMENTS / GOALS / SUPPLEMENTS USED

"Finally, be strong in the Lord and in His mighty power."
-Ephesians 6:10 (NIV)

DATE: _______   PLACE:____________________   WEIGHT:_______

EXERCISE		SET 1	SET 2	SET 3	SET 4	SET 5	SET 6	SET 7
SQUAT	REPS							
	WEIGHT							
BENCH PRESS	REPS							
	WEIGHT							
DEADLIFT	REPS							
	WEIGHT							
CURL	REPS							
	WEIGHT							

ASSISTANCE EXERCISES		SET 1	SET 2	SET 3	SET 4	SET 5
	REPS					
	WEIGHT					
	REPS					
	WEIGHT					
	REPS					
	WEIGHT					
	REPS					
	WEIGHT					

COMMENTS / GOALS / SUPPLEMENTS USED

"It's not the size of the dog in the fight, it's the size of the fight in the dog." –Mark Twain

DATE: _______   PLACE:_____________________   WEIGHT:_______

EXERCISE		SET 1	SET 2	SET 3	SET 4	SET 5	SET 6	SET 7
SQUAT	REPS							
	WEIGHT							
BENCH PRESS	REPS							
	WEIGHT							
DEADLIFT	REPS							
	WEIGHT							
CURL	REPS							
	WEIGHT							

ASSISTANCE EXERCISES		SET 1	SET 2	SET 3	SET 4	SET 5
	REPS					
	WEIGHT					
	REPS					
	WEIGHT					
	REPS					
	WEIGHT					
	REPS					
	WEIGHT					

COMMENTS / GOALS / SUPPLEMENTS USED

"Make every rep and every set count."
-Robert L. Dunn

DATE: _______   PLACE:____________________ WEIGHT:______

EXERCISE		SET 1	SET 2	SET 3	SET 4	SET 5	SET 6	SET 7
SQUAT	REPS							
	WEIGHT							
BENCH PRESS	REPS							
	WEIGHT							
DEADLIFT	REPS							
	WEIGHT							
CURL	REPS							
	WEIGHT							

ASSISTANCE EXERCISES		SET 1	SET 2	SET 3	SET 4	SET 5
	REPS					
	WEIGHT					
	REPS					
	WEIGHT					
	REPS					
	WEIGHT					
	REPS					
	WEIGHT					

COMMENTS / GOALS / SUPPLEMENTS USED

"When you are on your deathbed, what will you regret not doing?" – Robert L. Dunn

DATE: _______   PLACE:____________________   WEIGHT:_______

EXERCISE		SET 1	SET 2	SET 3	SET 4	SET 5	SET 6	SET 7
SQUAT	REPS							
	WEIGHT							
BENCH PRESS	REPS							
	WEIGHT							
DEADLIFT	REPS							
	WEIGHT							
CURL	REPS							
	WEIGHT							

ASSISTANCE EXERCISES		SET 1	SET 2	SET 3	SET 4	SET 5
	REPS					
	WEIGHT					
	REPS					
	WEIGHT					
	REPS					
	WEIGHT					
	REPS					
	WEIGHT					

COMMENTS / GOALS / SUPPLEMENTS USED

"Arriving at one goal is the starting point to another."
-John Dewey

DATE: _______   PLACE:____________________   WEIGHT:_______

EXERCISE		SET 1	SET 2	SET 3	SET 4	SET 5	SET 6	SET 7
SQUAT	REPS							
	WEIGHT							
BENCH PRESS	REPS							
	WEIGHT							
DEADLIFT	REPS							
	WEIGHT							
CURL	REPS							
	WEIGHT							

ASSISTANCE EXERCISES		SET 1	SET 2	SET 3	SET 4	SET 5
	REPS					
	WEIGHT					
	REPS					
	WEIGHT					
	REPS					
	WEIGHT					
	REPS					
	WEIGHT					

COMMENTS / GOALS / SUPPLEMENTS USED

"He who would arrive at the appointed end must follow a single road and not wander through many ways."
-Seneca

DATE: _______   PLACE:____________________ WEIGHT:_______

EXERCISE		SET 1	SET 2	SET 3	SET 4	SET 5	SET 6	SET 7
SQUAT	REPS							
	WEIGHT							
BENCH PRESS	REPS							
	WEIGHT							
DEADLIFT	REPS							
	WEIGHT							
CURL	REPS							
	WEIGHT							

ASSISTANCE EXERCISES		SET 1	SET 2	SET 3	SET 4	SET 5
	REPS					
	WEIGHT					
	REPS					
	WEIGHT					
	REPS					
	WEIGHT					
	REPS					
	WEIGHT					

COMMENTS / GOALS / SUPPLEMENTS USED

"Life can be pulled by goals just as surely as it can be pulled by drives." – Victor Frankl

DATE: _______   PLACE: ____________________   WEIGHT: _______

EXERCISE		SET 1	SET 2	SET 3	SET 4	SET 5	SET 6	SET 7
SQUAT	REPS							
	WEIGHT							
BENCH	REPS							
PRESS	WEIGHT							
DEADLIFT	REPS							
	WEIGHT							
CURL	REPS							
	WEIGHT							

ASSISTANCE EXERCISES	SET 1	SET 2	SET 3	SET 4	SET 5
REPS					
WEIGHT					
REPS					
WEIGHT					
REPS					
WEIGHT					
REPS					
WEIGHT					

COMMENTS / GOALS / SUPPLEMENTS USED

"The virtue lies in the struggle, not in the prize."
-Richard Monckton Milnes

DATE: _______   PLACE: _______________________   WEIGHT: _______

EXERCISE		SET 1	SET 2	SET 3	SET 4	SET 5	SET 6	SET 7
SQUAT	REPS							
	WEIGHT							
BENCH PRESS	REPS							
	WEIGHT							
DEADLIFT	REPS							
	WEIGHT							
CURL	REPS							
	WEIGHT							

ASSISTANCE EXERCISES		SET 1	SET 2	SET 3	SET 4	SET 5
	REPS					
	WEIGHT					
	REPS					
	WEIGHT					
	REPS					
	WEIGHT					
	REPS					
	WEIGHT					

COMMENTS / GOALS / SUPPLEMENTS USED

"The wolf on the hill is not as hungry as the wolf climbing the hill." -Unknown

DATE: _______   PLACE:____________________ WEIGHT:_______

EXERCISE		SET 1	SET 2	SET 3	SET 4	SET 5	SET 6	SET 7
SQUAT	REPS							
	WEIGHT							
BENCH	REPS							
PRESS	WEIGHT							
DEADLIFT	REPS							
	WEIGHT							
CURL	REPS							
	WEIGHT							

ASSISTANCE EXERCISES		SET 1	SET 2	SET 3	SET 4	SET 5
	REPS					
	WEIGHT					
	REPS					
	WEIGHT					
	REPS					
	WEIGHT					
	REPS					
	WEIGHT					

COMMENTS / GOALS / SUPPLEMENTS USED

*"It is better to fall short of a high mark
than to reach a low one." –H.C. Payne*

DATE: _______   PLACE:____________________ WEIGHT:_______

EXERCISE		SET 1	SET 2	SET 3	SET 4	SET 5	SET 6	SET 7
SQUAT	REPS							
	WEIGHT							
BENCH PRESS	REPS							
	WEIGHT							
DEADLIFT	REPS							
	WEIGHT							
CURL	REPS							
	WEIGHT							

ASSISTANCE EXERCISES		SET 1	SET 2	SET 3	SET 4	SET 5
	REPS					
	WEIGHT					
	REPS					
	WEIGHT					
	REPS					
	WEIGHT					
	REPS					
	WEIGHT					

COMMENTS / GOALS / SUPPLEMENTS USED

"With the day comes new strength and new thoughts."
-Eleanor Roosevelt

DATE: _______   PLACE:____________________   WEIGHT:_______

EXERCISE		SET 1	SET 2	SET 3	SET 4	SET 5	SET 6	SET 7
SQUAT	REPS							
	WEIGHT							
BENCH	REPS							
PRESS	WEIGHT							
DEADLIFT	REPS							
	WEIGHT							
CURL	REPS							
	WEIGHT							

ASSISTANCE EXERCISES		SET 1	SET 2	SET 3	SET 4	SET 5
	REPS					
	WEIGHT					
	REPS					
	WEIGHT					
	REPS					
	WEIGHT					
	REPS					
	WEIGHT					

COMMENTS / GOALS / SUPPLEMENTS USED

"Never take a day for granted. Start your bucket list today."
-Robert L. Dunn

DATE: _______ PLACE: __________________ WEIGHT:_______

EXERCISE		SET 1	SET 2	SET 3	SET 4	SET 5	SET 6	SET 7
SQUAT	REPS							
	WEIGHT							
BENCH PRESS	REPS							
	WEIGHT							
DEADLIFT	REPS							
	WEIGHT							
CURL	REPS							
	WEIGHT							

ASSISTANCE EXERCISES		SET 1	SET 2	SET 3	SET 4	SET 5
	REPS					
	WEIGHT					
	REPS					
	WEIGHT					
	REPS					
	WEIGHT					
	REPS					
	WEIGHT					

COMMENTS / GOALS / SUPPLEMENTS USED

"The past cannot be changed.
The future is yet in your power." -Unknown

DATE: _______   PLACE:____________________   WEIGHT:_______

EXERCISE		SET 1	SET 2	SET 3	SET 4	SET 5	SET 6	SET 7
SQUAT	REPS							
	WEIGHT							
BENCH PRESS	REPS							
	WEIGHT							
DEADLIFT	REPS							
	WEIGHT							
CURL	REPS							
	WEIGHT							

ASSISTANCE EXERCISES		SET 1	SET 2	SET 3	SET 4	SET 5
	REPS					
	WEIGHT					
	REPS					
	WEIGHT					
	REPS					
	WEIGHT					
	REPS					
	WEIGHT					

COMMENTS / GOALS / SUPPLEMENTS USED

"If you can dream it, you can do it."
-Walt Disney

DATE: _______ PLACE:____________________ WEIGHT:______

EXERCISE		SET 1	SET 2	SET 3	SET 4	SET 5	SET 6	SET 7
SQUAT	REPS							
	WEIGHT							
BENCH PRESS	REPS							
	WEIGHT							
DEADLIFT	REPS							
	WEIGHT							
CURL	REPS							
	WEIGHT							

ASSISTANCE EXERCISES		SET 1	SET 2	SET 3	SET 4	SET 5
	REPS					
	WEIGHT					
	REPS					
	WEIGHT					
	REPS					
	WEIGHT					
	REPS					
	WEIGHT					

COMMENTS / GOALS / SUPPLEMENTS USED

"The key is to keep company only with people who uplift you, whose presence calls forth your best."
-Epictetus

DATE: _______   PLACE:___________________   WEIGHT:_______

EXERCISE		SET 1	SET 2	SET 3	SET 4	SET 5	SET 6	SET 7
SQUAT	REPS							
	WEIGHT							
BENCH PRESS	REPS							
	WEIGHT							
DEADLIFT	REPS							
	WEIGHT							
CURL	REPS							
	WEIGHT							

ASSISTANCE EXERCISES		SET 1	SET 2	SET 3	SET 4	SET 5
	REPS					
	WEIGHT					
	REPS					
	WEIGHT					
	REPS					
	WEIGHT					
	REPS					
	WEIGHT					

COMMENTS / GOALS / SUPPLEMENTS USED

*"You cannot wait for inspiration,
you have to go after it with a club."* –Jack London

DATE: _______   PLACE:___________________   WEIGHT:_______

EXERCISE		SET 1	SET 2	SET 3	SET 4	SET 5	SET 6	SET 7
SQUAT	REPS							
	WEIGHT							
BENCH PRESS	REPS							
	WEIGHT							
DEADLIFT	REPS							
	WEIGHT							
CURL	REPS							
	WEIGHT							

ASSISTANCE EXERCISES		SET 1	SET 2	SET 3	SET 4	SET 5
	REPS					
	WEIGHT					
	REPS					
	WEIGHT					
	REPS					
	WEIGHT					
	REPS					
	WEIGHT					

COMMENTS / GOALS / SUPPLEMENTS USED

*"It's not whether you get knocked down;
it's whether you get up." –Vince Lombardi*

DATE: _______   PLACE: ______________________   WEIGHT: _______

EXERCISE		SET 1	SET 2	SET 3	SET 4	SET 5	SET 6	SET 7
SQUAT	REPS							
	WEIGHT							
BENCH PRESS	REPS							
	WEIGHT							
DEADLIFT	REPS							
	WEIGHT							
CURL	REPS							
	WEIGHT							

ASSISTANCE EXERCISES		SET 1	SET 2	SET 3	SET 4	SET 5
	REPS					
	WEIGHT					
	REPS					
	WEIGHT					
	REPS					
	WEIGHT					
	REPS					
	WEIGHT					

COMMENTS / GOALS / SUPPLEMENTS USED

"Nobody who gave his best has regretted it."
-George Halas

DATE: ________ PLACE:________________________ WEIGHT:_______

EXERCISE		SET 1	SET 2	SET 3	SET 4	SET 5	SET 6	SET 7
SQUAT	REPS							
	WEIGHT							
BENCH PRESS	REPS							
	WEIGHT							
DEADLIFT	REPS							
	WEIGHT							
CURL	REPS							
	WEIGHT							

ASSISTANCE EXERCISES		SET 1	SET 2	SET 3	SET 4	SET 5
	REPS					
	WEIGHT					
	REPS					
	WEIGHT					
	REPS					
	WEIGHT					
	REPS					
	WEIGHT					

COMMENTS / GOALS / SUPPLEMENTS USED

"Make sure your worst enemy doesn't live between your own two ears." –Laird Hamilton

DATE: _______   PLACE:_____________________   WEIGHT:_______

EXERCISE		SET 1	SET 2	SET 3	SET 4	SET 5	SET 6	SET 7
SQUAT	REPS							
	WEIGHT							
BENCH PRESS	REPS							
	WEIGHT							
DEADLIFT	REPS							
	WEIGHT							
CURL	REPS							
	WEIGHT							

ASSISTANCE EXERCISES		SET 1	SET 2	SET 3	SET 4	SET 5
	REPS					
	WEIGHT					
	REPS					
	WEIGHT					
	REPS					
	WEIGHT					
	REPS					
	WEIGHT					

COMMENTS / GOALS / SUPPLEMENTS USED

"The biggest failure you can have in life is making the mistake of never trying at all." -Unknown

DATE: ______ PLACE:____________________ WEIGHT:______

EXERCISE		SET 1	SET 2	SET 3	SET 4	SET 5	SET 6	SET 7
SQUAT	REPS							
	WEIGHT							
BENCH PRESS	REPS							
	WEIGHT							
DEADLIFT	REPS							
	WEIGHT							
CURL	REPS							
	WEIGHT							

ASSISTANCE EXERCISES		SET 1	SET 2	SET 3	SET 4	SET 5
	REPS					
	WEIGHT					
	REPS					
	WEIGHT					
	REPS					
	WEIGHT					
	REPS					
	WEIGHT					

COMMENTS / GOALS / SUPPLEMENTS USED

"Better to wear out than rust out."
-Jack LaLanne

DATE: _______   PLACE:_____________________   WEIGHT:_______

EXERCISE		SET 1	SET 2	SET 3	SET 4	SET 5	SET 6	SET 7
SQUAT	REPS							
	WEIGHT							
BENCH PRESS	REPS							
	WEIGHT							
DEADLIFT	REPS							
	WEIGHT							
CURL	REPS							
	WEIGHT							

ASSISTANCE EXERCISES		SET 1	SET 2	SET 3	SET 4	SET 5
	REPS					
	WEIGHT					
	REPS					
	WEIGHT					
	REPS					
	WEIGHT					
	REPS					
	WEIGHT					

COMMENTS / GOALS / SUPPLEMENTS USED

"Forget all the reasons it won't work and believe the one reason that it will." -Unknown

DATE: _______   PLACE:_____________________   WEIGHT:_______

EXERCISE		SET 1	SET 2	SET 3	SET 4	SET 5	SET 6	SET 7
SQUAT	REPS							
	WEIGHT							
BENCH PRESS	REPS							
	WEIGHT							
DEADLIFT	REPS							
	WEIGHT							
CURL	REPS							
	WEIGHT							

ASSISTANCE EXERCISES		SET 1	SET 2	SET 3	SET 4	SET 5
	REPS					
	WEIGHT					
	REPS					
	WEIGHT					
	REPS					
	WEIGHT					
	REPS					
	WEIGHT					

COMMENTS / GOALS / SUPPLEMENTS USED

"A journey of a thousand miles begins with a single step."
-Lao Tzu

DATE: _______   PLACE: ___________________   WEIGHT: _______

EXERCISE		SET 1	SET 2	SET 3	SET 4	SET 5	SET 6	SET 7
SQUAT	REPS							
	WEIGHT							
BENCH PRESS	REPS							
	WEIGHT							
DEADLIFT	REPS							
	WEIGHT							
CURL	REPS							
	WEIGHT							

ASSISTANCE EXERCISES		SET 1	SET 2	SET 3	SET 4	SET 5
	REPS					
	WEIGHT					
	REPS					
	WEIGHT					
	REPS					
	WEIGHT					
	REPS					
	WEIGHT					

COMMENTS / GOALS / SUPPLEMENTS USED

"You have power over your mind not outside events.
Realize this, and you will find strength."
–Marcus Aurelius

DATE: _______   PLACE:___________________   WEIGHT:_______

EXERCISE		SET 1	SET 2	SET 3	SET 4	SET 5	SET 6	SET 7
SQUAT	REPS							
	WEIGHT							
BENCH PRESS	REPS							
	WEIGHT							
DEADLIFT	REPS							
	WEIGHT							
CURL	REPS							
	WEIGHT							

ASSISTANCE EXERCISES		SET 1	SET 2	SET 3	SET 4	SET 5
	REPS					
	WEIGHT					
	REPS					
	WEIGHT					
	REPS					
	WEIGHT					
	REPS					
	WEIGHT					

COMMENTS / GOALS / SUPPLEMENTS USED

"I can do all things through him who strengthens me."
-Philippians 4:13 (ESV)

DATE: _______   PLACE:_____________________   WEIGHT:_______

EXERCISE		SET 1	SET 2	SET 3	SET 4	SET 5	SET 6	SET 7
SQUAT	REPS							
	WEIGHT							
BENCH	REPS							
PRESS	WEIGHT							
DEADLIFT	REPS							
	WEIGHT							
CURL	REPS							
	WEIGHT							

ASSISTANCE EXERCISES		SET 1	SET 2	SET 3	SET 4	SET 5
	REPS					
	WEIGHT					
	REPS					
	WEIGHT					
	REPS					
	WEIGHT					
	REPS					
	WEIGHT					

COMMENTS / GOALS / SUPPLEMENTS USED

"For the spirit God gave us does not make us timid, but gives us power, love and self-discipline." -2 Timothy 1:7 (NIV)

DATE: _______   PLACE:____________________ WEIGHT:_______

EXERCISE		SET 1	SET 2	SET 3	SET 4	SET 5	SET 6	SET 7
SQUAT	REPS							
	WEIGHT							
BENCH PRESS	REPS							
	WEIGHT							
DEADLIFT	REPS							
	WEIGHT							
CURL	REPS							
	WEIGHT							

ASSISTANCE EXERCISES		SET 1	SET 2	SET 3	SET 4	SET 5
	REPS					
	WEIGHT					
	REPS					
	WEIGHT					
	REPS					
	WEIGHT					
	REPS					
	WEIGHT					

COMMENTS / GOALS / SUPPLEMENTS USED

"Adversity causes some men to break;
others to break records." –William Ward

DATE: _______   PLACE: ___________________ WEIGHT: _______

EXERCISE		SET 1	SET 2	SET 3	SET 4	SET 5	SET 6	SET 7
SQUAT	REPS							
	WEIGHT							
BENCH PRESS	REPS							
	WEIGHT							
DEADLIFT	REPS							
	WEIGHT							
CURL	REPS							
	WEIGHT							

ASSISTANCE EXERCISES		SET 1	SET 2	SET 3	SET 4	SET 5
	REPS					
	WEIGHT					
	REPS					
	WEIGHT					
	REPS					
	WEIGHT					
	REPS					
	WEIGHT					

COMMENTS / GOALS / SUPPLEMENTS USED

"There are two ways to live your life. One is as nothing is a miracle. The other is as everything is miracle."
-Albert Einstein

DATE: _______   PLACE:____________________ WEIGHT:_______

EXERCISE		SET 1	SET 2	SET 3	SET 4	SET 5	SET 6	SET 7
SQUAT	REPS							
	WEIGHT							
BENCH PRESS	REPS							
	WEIGHT							
DEADLIFT	REPS							
	WEIGHT							
CURL	REPS							
	WEIGHT							

ASSISTANCE EXERCISES		SET 1	SET 2	SET 3	SET 4	SET 5
	REPS					
	WEIGHT					
	REPS					
	WEIGHT					
	REPS					
	WEIGHT					
	REPS					
	WEIGHT					

COMMENTS / GOALS / SUPPLEMENTS USED

"Optimism is the faith that leads to achievement."
-Helen Keller

DATE: _______   PLACE: _____________________ WEIGHT: _______

EXERCISE		SET 1	SET 2	SET 3	SET 4	SET 5	SET 6	SET 7
SQUAT	REPS							
	WEIGHT							
BENCH PRESS	REPS							
	WEIGHT							
DEADLIFT	REPS							
	WEIGHT							
CURL	REPS							
	WEIGHT							

ASSISTANCE EXERCISES		SET 1	SET 2	SET 3	SET 4	SET 5
	REPS					
	WEIGHT					
	REPS					
	WEIGHT					
	REPS					
	WEIGHT					
	REPS					
	WEIGHT					

COMMENTS / GOALS / SUPPLEMENTS USED

"Persistence can change failure into extraordinary achievement." –Matt Biondi

DATE: _______   PLACE:_____________________   WEIGHT:_______

EXERCISE		SET 1	SET 2	SET 3	SET 4	SET 5	SET 6	SET 7
SQUAT	REPS							
	WEIGHT							
BENCH PRESS	REPS							
	WEIGHT							
DEADLIFT	REPS							
	WEIGHT							
CURL	REPS							
	WEIGHT							

ASSISTANCE EXERCISES		SET 1	SET 2	SET 3	SET 4	SET 5
	REPS					
	WEIGHT					
	REPS					
	WEIGHT					
	REPS					
	WEIGHT					
	REPS					
	WEIGHT					

COMMENTS / GOALS / SUPPLEMENTS USED

"A goal is a dream with a deadline."
-Napoleon Hill

DATE: _______   PLACE: ___________________   WEIGHT: _______

EXERCISE		SET 1	SET 2	SET 3	SET 4	SET 5	SET 6	SET 7
SQUAT	REPS							
	WEIGHT							
BENCH PRESS	REPS							
	WEIGHT							
DEADLIFT	REPS							
	WEIGHT							
CURL	REPS							
	WEIGHT							

ASSISTANCE EXERCISES		SET 1	SET 2	SET 3	SET 4	SET 5
	REPS					
	WEIGHT					
	REPS					
	WEIGHT					
	REPS					
	WEIGHT					
	REPS					
	WEIGHT					

COMMENTS / GOALS / SUPPLEMENTS USED

*"Ah, but a man's reach should exceed his grasp,
or what's a heaven for?" –Robert Browning*

DATE: _______ PLACE:______________________ WEIGHT:_______

EXERCISE		SET 1	SET 2	SET 3	SET 4	SET 5	SET 6	SET 7
SQUAT	REPS							
	WEIGHT							
BENCH	REPS							
PRESS	WEIGHT							
DEADLIFT	REPS							
	WEIGHT							
CURL	REPS							
	WEIGHT							

ASSISTANCE EXERCISES		SET 1	SET 2	SET 3	SET 4	SET 5
	REPS					
	WEIGHT					
	REPS					
	WEIGHT					
	REPS					
	WEIGHT					
	REPS					
	WEIGHT					

COMMENTS / GOALS / SUPPLEMENTS USED

"Things won are done; joy's soul lies in the doing."
-William Shakespeare

DATE: _______ PLACE:___________________ WEIGHT:_______

EXERCISE		SET 1	SET 2	SET 3	SET 4	SET 5	SET 6	SET 7
SQUAT	REPS							
	WEIGHT							
BENCH PRESS	REPS							
	WEIGHT							
DEADLIFT	REPS							
	WEIGHT							
CURL	REPS							
	WEIGHT							

ASSISTANCE EXERCISES		SET 1	SET 2	SET 3	SET 4	SET 5
	REPS					
	WEIGHT					
	REPS					
	WEIGHT					
	REPS					
	WEIGHT					
	REPS					
	WEIGHT					

COMMENTS / GOALS / SUPPLEMENTS USED

"Dream more than others think practical.
Expect more than others think possible." –Frank Zane

DATE: _______ PLACE:____________________ WEIGHT:______

EXERCISE		SET 1	SET 2	SET 3	SET 4	SET 5	SET 6	SET 7
SQUAT	REPS							
	WEIGHT							
BENCH PRESS	REPS							
	WEIGHT							
DEADLIFT	REPS							
	WEIGHT							
CURL	REPS							
	WEIGHT							

ASSISTANCE EXERCISES		SET 1	SET 2	SET 3	SET 4	SET 5
	REPS					
	WEIGHT					
	REPS					
	WEIGHT					
	REPS					
	WEIGHT					
	REPS					
	WEIGHT					

COMMENTS / GOALS / SUPPLEMENTS USED

"Be of good courage, and he shall strengthen your heart, all ye that hope in the Lord." –Psalm 31:24 (KJV)

DATE: _______   PLACE:____________________ WEIGHT:_______

EXERCISE		SET 1	SET 2	SET 3	SET 4	SET 5	SET 6	SET 7
SQUAT	REPS							
	WEIGHT							
BENCH PRESS	REPS							
	WEIGHT							
DEADLIFT	REPS							
	WEIGHT							
CURL	REPS							
	WEIGHT							

ASSISTANCE EXERCISES		SET 1	SET 2	SET 3	SET 4	SET 5
	REPS					
	WEIGHT					
	REPS					
	WEIGHT					
	REPS					
	WEIGHT					
	REPS					
	WEIGHT					

COMMENTS / GOALS / SUPPLEMENTS USED

*"Not everyone will understand your journey. That's fine.
It's not their journey to make sense of. It's yours."*
–Zero Dean

DATE: _______   PLACE:____________________   WEIGHT:_______

EXERCISE		SET 1	SET 2	SET 3	SET 4	SET 5	SET 6	SET 7
SQUAT	REPS							
	WEIGHT							
BENCH	REPS							
PRESS	WEIGHT							
DEADLIFT	REPS							
	WEIGHT							
CURL	REPS							
	WEIGHT							

ASSISTANCE EXERCISES		SET 1	SET 2	SET 3	SET 4	SET 5
	REPS					
	WEIGHT					
	REPS					
	WEIGHT					
	REPS					
	WEIGHT					
	REPS					
	WEIGHT					

COMMENTS / GOALS / SUPPLEMENTS USED

"God opens many doors for you, how many will you close?"
-Robert L. Dunn

HOW TO DOCUMENT
WORKOUTS
IN THIS BOOK

SAMPLE WORKOUT 1:

DATE: <u>7/1/2018</u> PLACE: <u>HOME GYM</u>   WEIGHT: <u>214</u>

EXERCISE		SET 1	SET 2	SET 3	SET 4	SET 5	SET 6	SET 7
SQUAT	REPS	5	5	5	3	1		
	WEIGHT	135	185	225	275	295		
BENCH	REPS	5	5	5	3	1		
PRESS	WEIGHT	135	155	185	205	225		
DEADLIFT	REPS							
	WEIGHT							
CURL	REPS							
	WEIGHT							

ASSISTANCE EXERCISES		SET 1	SET 2	SET 3	SET 4	SET 5
DB	REPS	8	6	6		
INCLINES	WEIGHT	40	45	50		
MILITARY	REPS	8	6	6		
PRESS	WEIGHT	80	90	100		
	REPS					
	WEIGHT					
	REPS					
	WEIGHT					

COMMENTS / GOALS / SUPPLEMENTS USED
Good workout, taking daily multivitamin, magnesium,
Joint support supplement, goals 315 squat,
250 bench press

"The deadlift also serves as a way to train the mind to do things that are hard." –Mark Rippetoe

SAMPLE WORKOUT 2:

DATE: 8/1/2018 PLACE: HOME GYM   WEIGHT: 218

EXERCISE		SET 1	SET 2	SET 3	SET 4	SET 5	SET 6	SET 7
SQUAT	REPS							
	WEIGHT							
BENCH PRESS	REPS							
	WEIGHT							
DEADLIFT	REPS	5	5	5	3	3		
	WEIGHT	135	185	225	275	295		
CURL	REPS	5	5	3	3	6		
	WEIGHT	75	85	105	115	85		

ASSISTANCE EXERCISES		SET 1	SET 2	SET 3	SET 4	SET 5
DB INCLINES	REPS					
	WEIGHT					
MILITARY PRESS	REPS					
	WEIGHT					
HEX BAR (TRAP BAR)	REPS	5	5	3		
	WEIGHT	135	185	225		
BENT OVER ROWS	REPS	5	5	5		
	WEIGHT	115	135	135		

COMMENTS / GOALS / SUPPLEMENTS USED
Felt great today, continuing to use Creatine and
BCAA'S
GOALS-400 deadlift, 140 curl

"Your body can stand almost anything. It's your mind that you have to convince." -Unknown

<u>**SAMPLE CONTEST LOG:**</u>

CONTEST LOG

DATE: <u>12/12/2017</u>

EVENT: <u>NORTHCOAST CHAMPIONSHIPS</u> LOCATION: <u>Clv, Ohio</u>

WEIGHT: <u>215</u> WEIGHT CLASS: <u>220</u>   AGE GROUP: <u>60-64 Open</u>

ATTEMPTS	1	2	3	4
SQUAT	270	297.6	314.1	
BENCH PRESS	220.4	236.9	248	
DEADLIFT	347.2	363.7	380.2	
CURL	95.9	108	117.9	125.7

AWARDS: 2nd in Age Group Powerlifting, 1st in Age Group Push/Pull, 3rd in Open Powerlifting, 2nd in Open Push/Pull, 1st in Age Group Curl, 2nd in Open Curl

COMMENTS: completed all lifts except for 4th attempt curl which was a national record attempt. Did 3 warm-ups for each lift. Overall, a great meet, pleased with my performance.

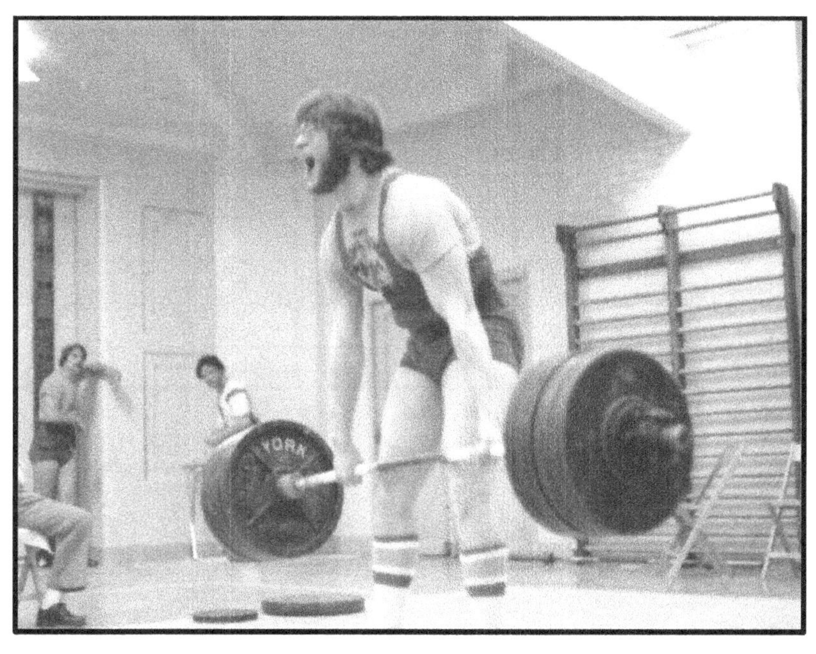

*"When my body SHOUTS stop,
my mind SCREAMS never."*
-Unknown

CONTEST LOG

DATE: ____________________

EVENT: _________________ **LOCATION:** ____________________

WEIGHT: _______ **WEIGHT CLASS:** ________ **AGE GROUP:** _________

ATTEMPTS	1	2	3	4
SQUAT				
BENCH PRESS				
DEADLIFT				
CURL				

AWARDS:
COMMENTS:

CONTEST LOG

DATE: ____________________

EVENT: _________________ **LOCATION:** ____________________

WEIGHT: _______ **WEIGHT CLASS:** ________ **AGE GROUP:** _________

ATTEMPTS	1	2	3	4
SQUAT				
BENCH PRESS				
DEADLIFT				
CURL				

AWARDS:
COMMENTS:

CONTEST LOG

DATE: _______________________

EVENT:_______________________ LOCATION:_______________________

WEIGHT:_______ WEIGHT CLASS:_________ AGE GROUP:___________

ATTEMPTS	1	2	3	4
SQUAT				
BENCH PRESS				
DEADLIFT				
CURL				

AWARDS:
COMMENTS:

CONTEST LOG

DATE: _______________________

EVENT:_______________________ LOCATION:_______________________

WEIGHT:_______ WEIGHT CLASS:_________ AGE GROUP:___________

ATTEMPTS	1	2	3	4
SQUAT				
BENCH PRESS				
DEADLIFT				
CURL				

AWARDS:
COMMENTS:

CONTEST LOG

DATE: _______________________

EVENT:_____________________ LOCATION:________________________

WEIGHT:_______ WEIGHT CLASS:________ AGE GROUP:__________

ATTEMPTS	1	2	3	4
SQUAT				
BENCH PRESS				
DEADLIFT				
CURL				

AWARDS:

COMMENTS:

CONTEST LOG

DATE: _______________________

EVENT:_____________________ LOCATION:________________________

WEIGHT:_______ WEIGHT CLASS:________ AGE GROUP:__________

ATTEMPTS	1	2	3	4
SQUAT				
BENCH PRESS				
DEADLIFT				
CURL				

AWARDS:

COMMENTS:

CONTEST LOG

DATE: _______________________

EVENT:___________________ LOCATION:______________________

WEIGHT:_______ WEIGHT CLASS:________ AGE GROUP:__________

ATTEMPTS	1	2	3	4
SQUAT				
BENCH PRESS				
DEADLIFT				
CURL				

AWARDS:
COMMENTS:

CONTEST LOG

DATE: _______________________

EVENT:___________________ LOCATION:______________________

WEIGHT:_______ WEIGHT CLASS:________ AGE GROUP:__________

ATTEMPTS	1	2	3	4
SQUAT				
BENCH PRESS				
DEADLIFT				
CURL				

AWARDS:
COMMENTS:

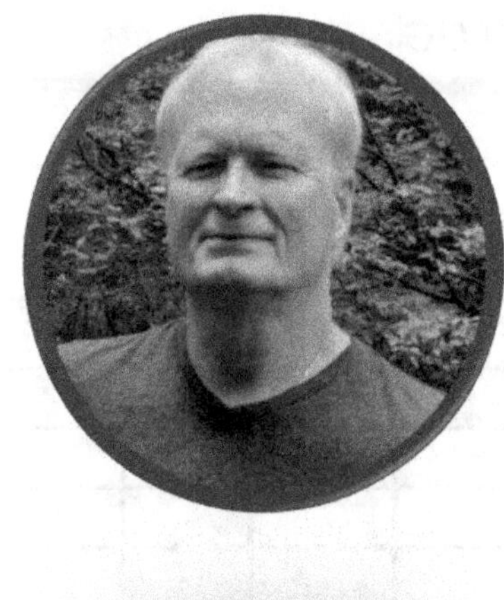

Robert Dunn is a Licensed Professional Clinical Counselor in the State of Ohio. He is a National Certified Counselor, a Master Addictions Counselor and an ACE Certified Personal Trainer. He holds Bachelors and Masters Degrees from Youngstown State University. He has extensive management and leadership experience and over thirty years of counseling and crisis intervention experience.

He is a published poet and has conducted seminars on a variety of mental health topics. He has done extensive research on anger, sports psychology, wellness, and mental health recovery. He provides outpatient counseling, anger management and wellness management and recovery groups at the Counseling Center at the Lisbon and Salem Ohio offices. Bob is a competitive powerlifter who regularly competes in 100% RAW Powerlifting Federation meets. He and his wife, Christine, have three adult children.

**OTHER BOOKS BY ROBERT L. DUNN
AVAILABLE FOR PURCHASE ON AMAZON:**

*68 Spiritual Solutions for Managing Anger

*The 8 Commandments of Anger Management

*Anger Management Guided Journal: A Path to Peace